YOUR KNOWLEDGE HAS VALUE

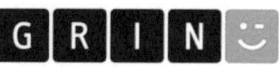

Amer A. Taqa, Nadira A. Hatim, Saja Amjad Abdul Razzak

Evaluate The Effect of Nigella Sativa and Thyme oil on the Color of Acrylic Resin Denture Base Material

GRIN Publishing

Bibliographic information published by the German National Library:

The German National Library lists this publication in the National Bibliography; detailed bibliographic data are available on the Internet at http://dnb.dnb.de .

Imprint:

Copyright © 2012 GRIN Verlag GmbH
Print and binding: Books on Demand GmbH, Norderstedt Germany
ISBN: 978-3-656-36417-7

This book at GRIN:

http://www.grin.com/en/e-book/207697/evaluate-the-effect-of-nigella-sativa-and-thyme-oil-on-the-color-of-acrylic

GRIN - Your knowledge has value

Since its foundation in 1998, GRIN has specialized in publishing academic texts by students, college teachers and other academics as e-book and printed book. The website www.grin.com is an ideal platform for presenting term papers, final papers, scientific essays, dissertations and specialist books.

Evaluate The Effect of *Nigella Sativa* and *Thyme* oil on the Color of Acrylic Resin Denture Base Material.

Running title: Color of Acrylic Resin Denture Base Material

Nadira A.Hatim	Dr.Amer A.Taqa	Saja Amjad Abdul Razzak
(Prof)	(Prof)	(Assit Lect)

Department of Prosthetic Dentistry

College of Dentistry, Mosul University

Abstract

The total number of samples (45) were divided into three main groups cured according to three curing cycles (The standard short cycle, rapid was subdivided into three subgroup: The control group (without additives), samples prepared with the addition of *Nigella Sativa* , and samples prepared with the addition of *Thyme* oil. Color was measured for all the samples. **Results** were analyzed statistically by (Descriptive statistics, ANOVA and Duncan's multiple range test) and showed that both additives(*Nigella Sativa* and *Thyme* oil) showed significant changes in the color of denture base. **conclusion** Both additives (*Nigella sativa* and *Thyme* oil) showed significant changes in the color of acrylic resin denture base material. The addition of *Thyme* oil to the samples cured by the regular heat curing cycle showed color change ($\Delta E=3.376$) in relation to the standard (ADA) cycle which is an acceptable range in vitro.

This study were to evaluate the effect of *Nigella sativa* and *Thyme* oil on The color of Acrylic Resin Denture Base Material.

Introduction

The number of denture wearers is increasing as the number of elderly people continually growing, and polymethylmethacrylate (PMMA) is still the most frequently used material in denture base fabrication[1].

Color stability is a required characteristic of denture base polymers, whether hard acrylic or soft lining materials, specified by various national and international standards typically as ADA specification No.12[2].

The color and translucency should be maintained during processing and these resins should not get stained or change in color through the clinical use. The color stability criteria may provide an important information on the service ability of the dental materials [3,4,5,6,7,8].

Various additives [(ethylene glycol dimethacrylate (EGDMA) [9],glass flake[10], rigid rod polymer (RRP) fillers[11], Chlorohexidine gluconate powder[12]] were added to acrylic resin to improve its flexural strength and modulous, microhardness, water sorption , solubility and flexibility.

Medical plant extracts (*Nigella sativa* and *Thyme* oil) were used as additives, as these oils were recommended to give suitable properties when added with certain concentrations on the heat cured acrylic resin [13,14]. Also these medical oils have antibacterial activity, *Nigella sativa* has greater effect, which may be due to the complex chemical structure of these seeds. These little seeds have over than one hundred different chemical components, including abundant sources of all the essential fatty acids, thougt that is often used medically. For example the essential oil of black cumin has an antimicrobial effect[15,16].

Materials and Methods

The total number of samples (45), were prepared from vertex heat cured denture base resin material according to manufacturer's instructions powder/liquid mixing ratio (2/1) . Samples were divided into three main groups:

1. The first group (15 samples) cured according to the standard short cycle[2] at 74 °C for 90 minutes, then at 100 °C for 30 minutes (5 samples were the control prepared without additives, 5 samples

prepared with the addition of *Nigella Sativa* oil and 5 samples prepared with the addition of *Thyme* oil).

2. The second group (15 samples) cured according to the standard rapid simplified manufacturer's instruction curing cycle at 70 °C for 10 minutes, then at 100 °C for 20 minutes (5 samples were the control prepared without additives, 5 samples prepared with the addition of *Nigella Sativa* oil and 5 samples prepared with the addition of *Thyme* oil).

3. The third group (15 samples) cured according to the standard regular manufacturer's instructions at 100 °C for 30 minutes (5 samples were the control prepared without additives, 5 samples prepared with the addition of *Nigella Sativa* oil and 5 samples prepared with the addition of *Thyme* oil).

The concentrations at which these additives added were 1.5% by weight[13]. The oil was added gradually (drop by drop) to the polymer with continuous mixing, then the monomer was added gradually to the mixture.

Note: The symbol (N) was added to the samples prepared with the addition of *Nigella sativa* and (T) for the samples prepared with the addition of *Thyme* oil.

1.Color Test (by the use of VITA Easyshade):

Acrylic samples were prepared with dimensions of (20x30x1.5) ± 0.03 mm[17]. Five samples were used for each group. After curing, the samples were stored in distilled water at 37 ± 1°C for 7 days before testing.

When the Easyshade device is warming up, the bottom of the screen displays a "presets" selection box. Touching "presets" allows Easyshade's default mode of operation to be selected and saved. This is achieved by the touch screen of the Easyshade.

The appropriate mode of measurement must be selected, and data reported are mode specific. In the measurements, "tooth single" mode of operation was selected and the device is adjusted to display the results of a measurement as L (Lightness), C (Chroma) and H (Hue).

The device must be calibrated each time when the unit was power – up, but not required between each measurement. Calibration is achieved by placing the 5 mm probe against a calibration block housed within the machine (Figure 1), according to the manufacturer's instructions.

The background color affects the color of denture base resins[18].So many trials were made to determine the standard method of color measurement of acrylic resin denture base material by using VITA Easyshade device.

1. Five samples of the standard short cycle (ADA) were measured with the presence of a white background .

2. The color of the above samples were measured without background and by placing additional samples of the same dimensions, starting by placing one by one and the number of additional samples was increased gradually until no change in measurements (lightness, chroma and hue) was detected and this is obtained by placing seven pieces under the measured sample .

3. Three edentulous patients with good oral health and normal color of the mucosa were selected and the above samples were measured intraorally on the three patients (the control method).

The results of color measurements (extraorally and intraorally) were statistically analyzed. It is shown that the measurements with one additional sample under the measured sample showed no significant difference from the intraoral measurements(Figure. 2,3,4). So this method was depended in this study for color measurements of all the samples .

(CIE L*a*b*) color difference metrics were used for the performance analysis of the samples in the current study. The measured values of L, C and H for each sample were transformed into baseline L*, a*, b* values. The total color change (ΔE) of each sample was calculated for each sample at each evaluation using the formula[19,20,21,22].:

$$\Delta E = [(\Delta L^*)^{2} + (\Delta a^*)^{2} + (\Delta b^*)^{2}]^{1/2}$$
$$\Delta E = [(L^*_2 - L^*_1)^{2} + (a^*_2 - a^*_1)^{2} + (b^*_2 - b^*_1)^{2}]^{1/2}$$

In principle, when no color difference will be detected after its exposure to the testing environment ($\Delta E=0$) [23]. ΔE of (3.7) or less is considered to be clinically acceptable in vitro study and of (6.8) is considered to be clinically acceptable in vivo study[23.20].

Results

Color Change Test

1.   By The Use of VITA Easyshade

It is shown from table (1) that there were significant changes in lightness, chroma and hue between the three standard curing cycles and their additive groups.

The number of samples, means, and standard deviations of the lightness, chroma and hue of the standard short cycle (S1), rapid simplified (MRa1), and regular heat curing (MRe1) cycles and samples cured according to these cycles with the addition of Nigella sativa and *Thyme* oil were shown in Tables (2), (3) and (4).

2. Measuring Color Changes According to the (CIE L* a* b*) Color System

It is shown from Table (5) that only *Thyme* oil additive when added to the samples of the standard regular heat curing cycle produced accepted color changes (in vitro) in comparison with its standard cycle and with the standard short cycle (ADA).

Discussion

Color Change:

It is shown from the results (Table 5) that the *Thyme* oil additive when added to the samples of the standard regular curing cycle, it would produce an accepted color change in vitro ($\Delta E=3.376$) in comparison with the standard short cycle (ADA) which is less than 3.7 which is considered as an acceptable range for color differences from the standard in vitro[23,20] .There were no previous studies to correlate these results with it.

Conclusion

1. Both additives (*Nigella sativa* and *Thyme* oil) showed significant changes in the color of acrylic resin denture base material.

2. The addition of *Thyme* oil to the samples cured by the regular heat curing cycle showed color change ($\Delta E=3.376$) in relation to the standard (ADA) cycle which is an acceptable range in vitro.

References

1. *Brown L.R., Flavin C., French H. Anew economy for a new century: State of the world. 1999, Cited in Ožen J., Sipahi C., Caglar A., Dalkiz M. In vitro cytotoxicity of glass and* carbon *Fiber – reinforced heat – polymerized acrylic resin denture base material.* **Turk J Med Sci.** *2005; 63: 121 – 126.*

2. *American Dental Association. Guide to dental materials and devices. 7th ed., Chicago.* **American Dental Association.** *1975; Pp. 203 – 208.*

3. *May K.B.,Razzoog M.E.,Koran A.,Robinson E. Denture base resin:Comparison study of color stability.* **J Prosthet Dent.** *1992; 68: 78– 82.*

4. *Beatty M.W., Mahanna G.K.,Bsie K.D., Jia W. Color change in dry-pigmented maxillofacial elastomer resulting from ultraviolet light exposure.* **J Prosthet Dent.** *1995 ; 74: 493– 498.*

5. *Lemon J.C.,Chambers M.S.,Jacobsen M.L.,Powers J.M. Color stability of facial prosthesis.* **J.Prosthet. Dent.** *1995; 74:613-*

618.

6. *Setz J.,Engel E.* In *Vitro color stability of resin veneered teltscopic denture.A double blind pilot study.* **J Prosthet Dent.** *1997; 77: 486 – 490.*

7. *Beatty M.W.,Mahanna G.K. Ultraviolet radiation-induced for color shifts occurring in oil-pigmented maxillofacial elastomer.* **J .Prosthet.Dent.** *1999; 82:441-446.*

8. *Polyzois G.L.,Yannikakis S.A.,Zissis A.J., Demertrion P.P. Color change of denture base materials after disinfection and sterilization immersion.* **Int.J.Prosthodont.** *1997; 10(1): 83-89.*

9. *Arima T., Hamada T., Mc cabe J.F. The effects of cross linking agents on some properties of HEMA-based resins.* **J Dent Res.** *1995; 9: 1597-1601.*

10. *Franklin P., Wood D.J., Bubb N.L. Reinforecement of poly(methyl methacrylate) denture base with glass flake.* **Dent. Mater.** *2005; 21:365-370.*

11. *Vuorinen A., Dyer S.R., Lassila L.V.G., Vallitu P.K. Effect of rigid rod polymer filler on mechanical properties of poly-methylmethacrylate denture base material.* **Dent Mater.** *2008; 24:708-713.*

12. *Taqa A.A., Mohammed N.Z., Alomari A.W. The Effect of addition Chlorhexidine Gluconate(powder) on the properties of heat cured acrylic resin. .* **Al – Rafidain Dent J.** *(5th scientific conference of dentistry college).2011;special issue:25-34.*

13. *Hatim N.A., Taqa A.A., Abbas W, Shuker A.M. The Effect of Thyme and Nigella oil on some properties of Acrylic Resin Denture Base .* **Al – Rafidain Dent J.** *2009;10(2):205-213.*

14. *Mohammed N.Z. The Effect of Thickness of Heat Cured Acrylic Resin with Additives on Water Sorption and Solubility.* **Al – Rafidain Dent J.** *2008;10(1):169-175.*

15. *Hamiton P. Learn the benefits of blackseed oil, but avoid cheap Nigella Sativa oil.* **Article Alley.***2007;June.*

16. *Cavar S., Maksimovic M., Solic M.E.,Jerkovic-Mujkic A.,Besta R.*

Chemical composition and antioxidant and antimicrobial activity of two Satureja essential oils.**Food chemicals.** *2008;111(3):648-653.*

17. Hatim N.A., Taqa A.A., Hasan R.H. Evaluation of the effect of curing techniques on color property of acrylic resins. **Al – Rafidain Dent J.** *2004; 4: 28 – 33.*

18. Powers J.M. and Lepeak P.J. Parameters that affect the color of denture resins. **J Dent Res.** *1977;11:1331-1335.*

19. Hersek N., Canay S., Uzun G., Yildiz F. Color stability of denture base acrylic resins in three food colorants. **J Prosthet Dent.** *1999; 81: 375 – 379.*

20. Alvin G.W., Delwin T.L., Shanglun K., William M.J. Color accuracy of commercial digital cameras for use in dentistry. **J oral rehabil.** *2006;22:553-559.*

21. Cal E., Guneri P., Kose T. Digital analysis , staining of mouth rinses characteristics on provisional acrylic resin. **J Oral Rehabil.** *2007;34:297-303.*

22. Anand M., Shetty P., Bhat S.G. Shade matching in fixed prosthodontics using instrumental color measurements and computers. **J Indian.Prothodont.society.***2007; 7: 179-183.*

23. Arthur S.K., Frederik C.S., John C. Color stability of provisional prosthodontic materials. **J Prosthet Dent.** *2004; 91:447-452.*

Table (1) The one way analysis of variance (ANOVA) for the Lightness, Chroma and Hue of the three standard curing cycles and their additive groups.

		Sum of squares	df	Mean square	F	Sig.
Lightness	Between groups	923.182	8	115.398	7.993	0.000*
	Within groups	519.728	36	14.437		
	Total	1442.910	44			
Chroma	Between groups	400.840	8	50.105	42.310	0.000*
	Within groups	42.632	36	1.184		
	Total	443.472	44			
Hue	Between groups	1216.416	8	152.052	227.169	0.000*
	Within groups	24.096	36	0.669		
	Total	1240.512	44			

* Significant difference at $p < 0.05$. df: Degree of freedom.

Table (2) Descriptive statistics of color change test measured by VITA Easyshade for the standard short cycle S1 (ADA) and its additive groups.

English Researches

Groups		N	Mean	Standard deviation	Minimum	Maximum
S1	**L**	5	63.780	0.383	63.5	64.4
	C	5	29.400	0.685	28.7	30.5
	H	5	46.940	0.409	46.4	47.3
S1N	**L**	5	67.960	1.281	66.1	69.7
	C	5	36.560	1.641	34.6	38.7
	H	5	52.820	1.971	51.0	55.5
S1T	**L**	5	58.800	1.391	56.6	60.3
	C	5	29.020	1.949	25.8	30.8
	H	5	42.560	0.114	42.4	42.7

N: Number of samples, L: Lightness, C: Chroma, H: Hue.

Table (3) Descriptive statistics of color change test measured by VITA Easyshade for the standard rapid simplified cycle and its additive groups

Groups		N	Mean	Standard deviation	Minimum	Maximum
MRa1	L	5	65.860	1.443	63.9	67.6
	C	5	29.860	0.687	29.0	30.7
	H	5	47.040	0.887	46.0	48.4
MRa1N	L	5	74.380	1.443	72.4	76.1
	C	5	35.080	0.589	34.5	35.8
	H	5	53.340	0.167	53.2	53.6
MRa1T	L	5	61.100	0.339	60.8	61.6
	C	5	34.220	0.449	33.8	34.8
	H	5	42.400	0.331	42.1	42.8

N: Number of samples, L: Lightness, C: Chroma, H: Hue.

Table (4) Descriptive statistics of color change test measured by VITA Easyshade among the standard regular heat curing cycle and its additive groups

Groups		N	Mean	Standard deviation	Minimum	Maximum
MRe1	L	5	63.740	0.482	63.3	64.4
	C	5	29.520	0.645	29.0	30.6
	H	5	46.640	0.251	46.4	47.0
MRe1N	L	5	70.480	1.035	69.7	72.3
	C	5	35.780	1.255	33.7	36.9
	H	5	58.780	0.668	57.6	59.2
MRe1T	L	5	63.380	0.476	62.8	64.0
	C	5	34.980	0.822	33.9	36.1
	H	5	44.600	0.721	43.6	45.3

N: Number of samples, L: Lightness, C: Chroma, H: Hue.

Table (5) Colour change of the three standard curing cycles and their additive groups.

Groups	ΔE	In vitro
S1 vs S1N	10.433	Not
S1 vs S1T	5.646	Not
MRa1 vs MRa1N	12.988	Not
MRa1 vs MRa1T	6.148	Not
S1 vs MRa1N	15.021	Not
S1 vs MRa1T	4.294	Not
MRe1 vs MRe1N	15.698	Not
MRe1 vs MRe1T	3.382	Accepted
S1 vs MRe1N	15.334	Not
S1 vs MRe1T	3.376	Accepted

$\Delta E = 0$ No change in color, $\Delta E \leq 3.7$ Change in color accepted in vitro.

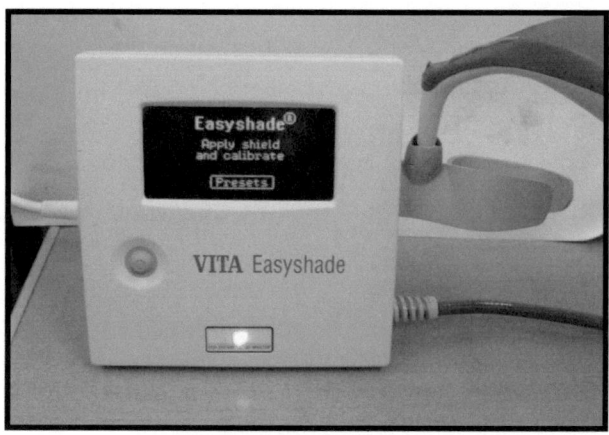

Figure (1): Calibration of the device.

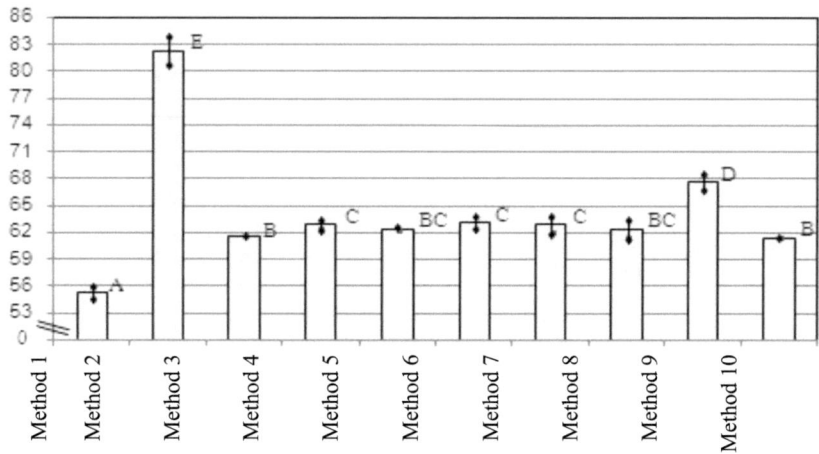

Figure (2): Mean ± SD and Duncan's Multiple Range Test for lightness
of the methods used in the pilot study of color measurement
by VITA Easyshade

* Different letters mean significant difference at $p \leq 0.05$, SD:Standard
Deviation.

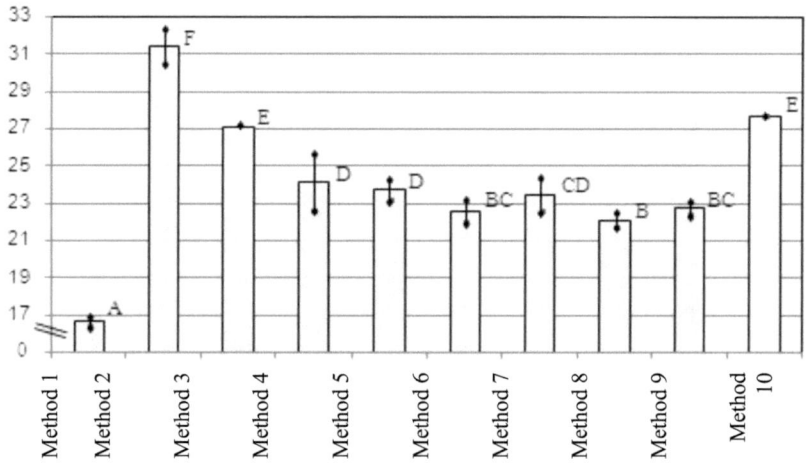

Figure (3): Mean ± SD and Duncan's Multiple Range Test for chroma of
the methods used in the pilot study of color measurement
by VITA Easyshade

* Different letters mean significant difference at $p \leq 0.05$, SD:Standard Deviation.

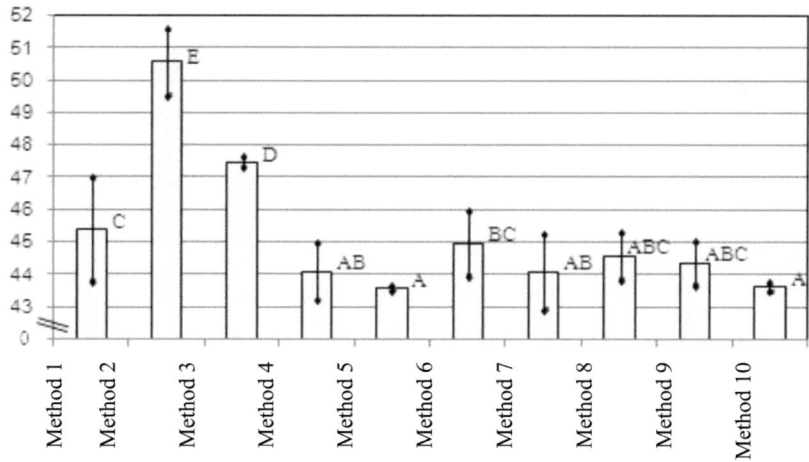

Figure (4): Mean $\pm$ SD and Duncan's Multiple Range Test for hue of the methods used in the pilot study of color measurement by VITA Easyshade

* Different letters mean significant difference at $p \leq 0.05$, SD:Stan.